HEALTHY EDUCATION HEALTHY LIFE TO LOSE WEIGHT

The vitamins and minerals in our body and the advantages of consuming them with diets.

JONATHAN VERA

ISBN: 9798634693026

DEDICATION

For all those people who lead or want to lead a healthy life.

You have wondered why some people look relatively young despite knowing their age and you realize from their physique they could look up to 10 years younger.

This book will teach you how to have a more balanced diet and how to get excellent results with vitamins and minerals.

CONTENTS

ACKNOWLEDGMENTS

Treat your body like a temple and not a garbage dump. Your body must be a good support system for the mind and spirit. If you CARE enough, your body can take you wherever you want to go, with the power, strength, energy and vitality you will need to get there.

Jim Rohn

1. THE VITAMINS

Vitamins are necessary for nutrients, the good cellular function of the body and, unlike some minerals; they act in very small doses. As our body cannot manufacture them by itself, the nutritional content of food could not be exploited since they activate the oxidation of food, metabolic operations and facilitate the use and release of energy provided through food.

Some vitamins are part of these enzymes, making them essential for body function. Of the 13 different vitamins that are currently known, we can differentiate two different groups:

1) WATER-SOLUBLE VITAMINS:

- Vitamin C - Ascorbic Acid
- Complex B
- Vitamin B 1 - Thiamine
- VitaminB2 - Riboflavin
- Vitamin B 3 - Niacin
- Vitamin B 5 - Pantothenic Acid
- Vitamin B6 - Pyridoxal
- Vitamin B 8- Biotin
- Vit. B12 - Cobalamin
- Folic Acid

2) **LIPOSOLUBLE VITAMINS:**

They dissolve in fats such as vitamins A, D, E, K. these are storeden adipose and liver tissues differ from water-soluble.

Excess consumption can be very harmful to health, since our body does store its excess. Both the lack and excess of some of them can cause irreversible diseases.

Soluble Vitamins

- Vitamin A – retinol
- Vitamin D 3 – calcitriol
- Vitamin E Vitamin E - α-tocopherol tocopherol
- Vitamin K – menaquinone

VITAMIN A
Function: helps growth and vision. Deficiency: decreased vision in dim light, dry skin, itchy eyes, and brittle nails.
Sources: butter, green leafy vegetables, spinach, fruits such as apricots, cod liver oil, eggs, milk, and carrots.

VITAMIN D
Function: together with vitamin A, it allows the absorption of Ca, it is essential for growth and calcification.
Deficiency: decalcification, rickets.

VITAMIN E

Function: facilitates blood circulation, and stabilizes female hormones, promoting pregnancy and childbirth.
Deficiency: anemia in premature infants.
Sources: nuts, eggs, butter, asparagus, spinach, and beans.

VITAMIN K

Function: acts on coagulation.
Deficiency: disturbances in blood coagulation.

Sources: potatoes, cauliflower, green beans, fresh peas and spinach. Liver, dairy products, eggs, sunlight, whose ultraviolet rays favor the absorption and assimilation of pro vitamins in vitamin D.

WATER-SOLUBLE VITAMINS: VITAMIN B1 or TIAMINE

Function: release energy that contains carbohydrates.
Deficiency: lowers blood glucose, fatigue, and irritability, and muscle weakness, lack of concentration or will.

Sources: nuts, whole grains, legumes, brewer's yeast and wheat germ.

VITAMIN B2 OR RIBOFLAVINE

Function: catalyze the oxidation of fats, proteins and carbohydrates.

Deficiency: visual disturbances, inflammation of the oral mucosa and throat.
Sources: liver, milk, beans, lentils, cheeses and nuts.

VITAMIN B3 NIACINE OR NICOTINIC ACID

Function: converting food energy is involved in the oxidation of carbohydrates and fatty acids.

Deficiency: produces Pellagra.

Sources: legumes, nuts, cereals, brewer's yeast.

VITAMIN B6 OR PYRIDOXINE

Function: metabolism of / amino acids and formation of hemoglobin.

Deficiency: does not seem to have a greater incidence on dietary problems.

Sources: bananas, avocados, whole grains, vegetables in general.

VITAMIN B9, M, FOLIC ACID OR FOLACINE

Function: it intervenes in the synthesis of DNA in the cells of new tissues, as is the case of fetuses; it also intervenes in the formation of red blood cells.

Deficiency: the lack of this vitamin induces a type of anemia that prevents the growth of red blood cells.

Sources: lentils, beans, vegetables, liver.

VITAMIN B12 OR CYANOCOBALAMINE:
Function: formation of red blood cells.

Deficiency: damage to nerve cells and pernicious anemia.

Sources: liver. It is the only vitamin that has a molecule with mineral, cobalt, and it is not produced by any plant or animal, but only by some microorganisms.

VITAMIN C OR ASCORBIC ACID

Function: formation of the protein of the connective tissues and regeneration of the cartilage of the bones.

Deficiency: connective tissue openings, subcutaneous hemorrhages, difficulty in healing of fractures or tooth loss.

Sources: potatoes, raw vegetables, citrus fruits, tomatoes, peppers, spinach.

VITAMIN H OR BIOTINE

Found in many plant and animal foods, so they do not usually offer dietary problems.

Source: beef and pork liver, egg yolk, spinach, brewer's yeast.

PANTOTHENIC ACID:

Function: defense of the organism against infections, it intervenes in the metabolism of fats, protein and carbohydrates.

Deficiency: lowers defenses against infection.

Sources: it is in all animal and plant tissues, beer yeast.

QUANTITY OR QUALITY?

Food is increasingly purified, refined and industrialized with treatments that improve preservation; the natural state of vitamins is altered and when they arrive at our table they have lost much of their nutritional value. Dietary imbalances such as junk food jump times, low calorie diets, produce a decrease in vitamins.

Other times, deficiencies are related to the use of chemical fertilizers instead of animal fertilizers. As nutrients in the body, vitamins are essential for life. The best way to consume them is natural and according to the variation depending on the vitamin content.

Sources: potatoes, raw vegetables, citrus fruits, tomatoes, peppers, spinach

VITAMIN H OR BIOTINE:

It is found in many plant and animal foods, so it does not usually offer dietary problems. Source: beef and pork liver, egg yolk, spinach, brewer's yeast.

PANTOTHENIC ACID:

Function: defense of the organism against infections, it intervenes in the metabolism of fats, protein and carbohydrates.

Deficiency: lowers defenses against infection. Sources: is in all animal and plant tissues, brewer's yeast

2. MINERALS

MINERALS. WHAT ARE THEY?

They are inorganic chemical elements. Also known as trace elements; and, although they are needed in small quantities, they are essential for the maintenance of life, growth and reproduction.

 What are the main minerals? What function do they have in our body? What happens if we are missing?

Zinc

Function: participates in the proper functioning of blood vessels and skin, nails and hair.

Natural source: meat, eggs, seafood and cereals. In walnuts, almonds, pumpkin seeds and popcorn.

Risk of deficit in vegetarians and prolonged diarrhea and malnutrition causing growth retardation, alopecia, skin and mucosa involvement.

Copper

Function: helps bone mineralization is an antioxidant and anti-inflammatory.

Natural source: liver, seafood, vegetables, nuts and seeds.

Deficit: due to insufficient intake or losses such as chronic diarrhea, burns and malnutrition.

Yodo

Function: it is necessary for the functioning of the thyroid.

Natural source: shellfish, fish, salmon, sardines, prawns, clams and mackerel. Pineapple.

Deficit: growth retardation and mental deficit.

Selenium

Function: antioxidant and for the proper functioning of the thyroid.

Natural source: cereals, meat, molluscs, fish, eggs and milk.

Deficit: in children fed prolonged parenteral nutrition, kidney or liver failure, or digestive malabsorption

Chrome

Function: it intervenes in the metabolism of sugars.

Natural source: meat, cereals, legumes, cheese, wheat germ, nuts and brewer's yeast.

Iron

Function: transport of oxygen to the cells.

Source: Food iron is used irregularly, but the intake of animal proteins (turkey, chicken, fish, legumes, clams, mussels, red meat) and vitamin C, help to increase absorption. The iron contained in whole grains, legumes, spinach is absorbed worse and its absorption improves if we combine them with foods rich in vitamin C such as kiwi, tomato, broccoli, orange, etc. Breast milk is low in iron but is compensated by its absorption, which is very high.

Deficit: It is frequent. In women due to menstrual losses and in pregnant women due to the high needs of the fetus, which may cause anemia. In children younger than two years (6-24 months) there is also a risk of anemia because iron needs are greater and the diet is still limited. It may be needed by babies exclusively breastfed beyond the 6th month or those who drink cow's milk before one year of age.

Fluorine

Function: it intervenes in the development and maintenance of teeth and bones.

Natural source: sea water, drinking water. Vegetables, meat, canned and smoked fish, seafood and tea. Toothpastes.

Deficit: dental caries. Tooth brushing with fluoride toothpastes should be performed (<500 ppm in children aged 2-6 and between 1000-1450 ppm in those over 6 years)

Calcium

Function: it intervenes in the nervous conduction, muscular contraction and in the maintenance of bones and teeth.

Natural source: dairy products (greater availability in breast milk than in infant formulas), nuts, legumes, meats. Calcium absorption improves with vitamin D and phosphorus...

Deficit: deformity in the skeleton of the child and adult, osteoporosis.

Magnesium

Function: skeletal and soft tissue formation. It prevents dental caries.

Natural source: seeds, vegetables, vegetables and to a lesser extent, milk, nuts, chocolate, banana, meat and fish.

Deficit: in digestive malabsorption, prolonged vomiting and diarrhea, kidney problems, etc.

When are vitamin supplements necessary?

The pediatrician will indicate when it is necessary for your child to take vitamin and / or mineral supplements. In case of strict vegetarian diets it may be necessary to supplement with Vitamin B12.

- In fat-free diets vitamins A, D and E will be supplemented.

- Children aged 1-3 years on diets without milk should receive calcium, vitamin D and riboflavin.

- Prematurity, pregnancy, lactation or adolescence are conditions in which the demand for minerals and vitamins increases and, in certain conditions, they can benefit from a vitamin / mineral supplement.

- There are chronic diseases that cause nutrient malabsorption, such as cystic fibrosis or celiac disease, and may require supplements.

Supplements are never a substitute for a balanced diet. If the child is a poor eater, the first thing to change is eating habits and behavior, and if necessary, due to little gain or loss of weight and height, your pediatrician will indicate the need to receive supplements.

Can they be dangerous?

Polyvitamin supplements may interact between their components with some medications.

The excess of vitamins can create dependency and appear adverse effects as a consequence of the excess of vitamins in the body.

They can cause allergic reactions.

Therefore, it should be studied if there is any vitamin and / or mineral deficiency and supplement the one that is exclusively necessary.

What are the daily needs of vitamins and minerals?

They are variable and with very wide margins depending on the age of the child, but with a varied diet they are easily met.

Final recommendations:

To ensure the necessary supply of vitamins and minerals we must:

- Consume two glasses of milk a day and complete with other dairy products.

- Take 3 servings of fruit a day and better without peeling.

- Take 2 servings of vegetables a day and undercooked.

- Consume all kinds of meat and fish with an average of 60 gr daily.

- Consume legumes twice a week.

- Maintain exclusive breastfeeding until the sixth month and thereafter introduce fruit and vegetable puree with meat and fish that cover the increased needs of vitamins and minerals.

- Favor daily sun exposure of at least 10 minutes a day.

When the diet is correct at each stage of life, the use of vitamin and mineral supplements can be avoided, unless there is a condition that suggests otherwise. Consuming a complete, balanced, adequate, innocuous, sufficient and varied diet will help maintain an optimal state of health and prevent diseases.

What is a vitamin and mineral supplement?

A vitamin and mineral supplement provides a variety of nutrients that are also found in food. These supplements are often called multivitamins. They come in the form of pills, chewable tablets, powders, and liquid.

A standard multivitamin usually contains:

• Vitamins soluble in water. These vitamins enter and leave the body with ease. Most do not accumulate in the cells of the body. Water soluble vitamins include vitamin C and B vitamins: thiamine, riboflavin, niacin, pantothenic acid, vitamin B6, biotin, folic acid, and vitamin B12.

• Fat soluble vitamins (fat soluble). These vitamins are stored in the body's cells and do not leave the body as easily as water soluble vitamins do. Fat-soluble vitamins include vitamins A, D, E, and K.

• Minerals. These include calcium, copper, iron, magnesium, phosphorous, potassium, selenium, and zinc.

Some multivitamins also contain other ingredients that are not vitamins or minerals. These include substances like the antioxidants lutein and lycopene.

Why take a supplement?

The best way to get the vitamins and minerals you need is to eat a wide variety of healthy foods. The Dietary Guidelines for Americans recommend fruits, vegetables, whole grains, milk and dairy products, and fish as part of a nutritional eating plan. A supplement cannot compensate for bad eating habits. But sometimes even people with healthy eating habits find it difficult to eat all the fruits, vegetables, and other healthy foods they need. A supplement can help make up for deficiencies.

Certain people are more likely to need a supplement. These include:

• People who eat a calorie restricted diet, which does not offer enough vitamins and minerals.

• Women who are pregnant or breastfeeding.

• People who are sick, injured, or recovering from surgery.

• Babies, especially to make sure they are getting the right amounts of calcium and vitamin D.

• People who are unable or unwilling to eat a variety of foods, such as people who have food allergies or those who follow a vegetarian diet.

What about supplements that are labeled for certain people (like women or the elderly)?

Many supplements are advertised as specially designed for men or women or for certain age groups. A standard multivitamin is appropriate for most people who take a supplement. But some people prefer to take a supplement that is made for their sex or age group.

The types of specialized supplements include:

• Formulas for women. Supplements for women have additional iron. This is because women who still have menstrual periods need more iron than men. But after menopause, women's iron needs are the same as men's.

Some formulas for women also contain additional calcium, since women are more likely to have osteoporosis than men.

• Formulas for men. These have a lower iron content, since men need less iron than women.

• Formulas for older adults. These are made for older adults and usually have less iron and vitamin K, and more vitamin B12 and vitamin D.

• Prenatal formulas. These are made for women who are pregnant, planning to become pregnant, or who are breastfeeding. Supplements have additional folic acid and iron. Folic acid is especially important because it can help prevent certain birth defects, especially birth defects of the neural tube. Sometimes these supplements also have more calcium.

What should you look for when choosing a supplement?

• Choose one that gives you a variety of vitamins and minerals (a multivitamin) instead of a supplement that gives you a single vitamin or mineral (unless your doctor has recommended that you take a single vitamin or single mineral).

• Choose the one that, along with the foods you eat, provides the recommended dietary allowance (RDA) for each vitamin and mineral. Supplements that provide much more than RDA can cause health problems. This is especially important for the minerals and fat soluble vitamins A, D, E and K. These are more easily stored in the body, and can accumulate to dangerous levels.

• Check the expiration date. Don't buy supplements that are expired or will expire before you can finish the bottle.

• If the supplement has the seal of the United States Pharmacopeia (USP), the supplement has been tested and contains the amounts of vitamins and minerals that are listed on the label.

• Check other ingredients on the label. Some supplements may contain food ingredients, such as wheat, corn, eggs, or gelatin. If you have a food allergy or are sensitive to these foods, look for supplements that don't have these ingredients.

A correct diet is key to ward off fatigue and tiredness, or often frequent ailments such as anemia (which is associated with a deficit of iron -one of the essential minerals for the functioning of our body-). That is why minerals and vitamins cannot be lacking in our diet; since these micronutrients are synonyms of health. So, you know, if you feel tired and need to build up your strength to get through the day, take a look at these highly nutritious foods!

Liver

One of the foods richest in iron and, therefore, essential to prevent and combat anemia, a disease that causes a decrease in red blood cells in the blood. However, while it is a very nutritious food, it also has its contraindications. On the one hand, it is a food that provides us with all kinds of vitamins -especially A, C, B and D.

And in case of anemia (very common in women athletes) it is the best option for its high absorption of iron. The problem is that the viscera, which, like in our body, acts as a filter for all kinds of substances, can be contaminated by heavy metals or other toxins.

Orange

All fruits are rich in vitamins, minerals, fiber and water, but citrus fruits are especially rich in vitamin C, key to the proper absorption of non-heme iron (the iron found in plant foods), which, like itself It is not well absorbed in our body, if we provide vitamin C before eating, it will help us absorb it. For example, drink orange juice before lentils. It also participates in the synthesis of neurotransmitters, avoiding fatigue, weakness and vasomotor instability. It is recommended not to replace processed fruits, such as canned or dried ones, with raw ones since they do not contain as many vitamins.

Spinach, broccoli, kale, and other leafy green vegetables.

We all know that we must incorporate vegetables into our daily diet, both raw and cooked. Its content in vitamins such as C is indisputable and in minerals such as potassium, so important in our body. Furthermore, they are very rich in antioxidants and have alkalizing properties. To preserve its vitamin content, the ideal is to consume it raw and, if cooking, better steamed. Always take advantage of the cooking broth to make soups, for example, since it maintains a large part of its vitamins.

Spices

Iron is also a mineral found in spices such as thyme, oregano and bay leaf. In addition to using them in the kitchen, they can be taken as infusions throughout the day.

Bread and whole grains

It is considered a complete food because it contains all the nutrients we need: protein, complex carbohydrates, 'good'

fats, vitamins, minerals and fiber.

Chocolate and cocoa

As it has been shown, chocolate has excellent properties, what is recommended is that 70% cocoa chocolate be consumed in order to take advantage of its benefits. It is very nutritious and rich in antioxidants, helping us in the prevention of cancer and cardiovascular disease. Dark chocolate lowers cholesterol levels, specifically LDL, that is, the bad one, and helps us against hypertension. It is also ideal for keeping skin nourished and hydrated.

Dairy products

They are a good source of vitamins and minerals such as calcium, an important mineral for maintaining bone mass. Milk and eggs are also rich in vitamin B12 - their deficiency is often associated with some types of anemia.

Walnuts

Nuts, especially walnuts, almonds, pistachios and sunflower seeds, can contribute up to 4 mg of iron per 100. A good way to include them in the diet is as a snack between meals.

Beer yeast

According to the nutrition expert and collaborator of Hello! In Shape, Marta Lorenzo is the most nutritious product or dietary supplement of all. It recommends us to include it in the diet daily for its high content of vitamins, mainly group B; in addition to containing essential amino acids and minerals such as potassium, selenium and phosphorus. Its benefits: it helps cellular restoration, strengthening our hair, nails and skin; promotes the proper functioning of the heart and liver, improves digestion and feeds our intestinal flora.

Rabbit

Rabbit meat is ideal for people who play sports, it is nutritious, high in protein, and low in fat.

3. OMEGAS

THE OMEGAS

When we talk about Omega 3, 6 or 9 we are not talking about a single compound but about families of similar fatty acids in chemical structure and biological function that, from the chemical point of view, are grouped according to the position in which the first double appears $C = C$ bond in its structure. Omega 3 and 6 cannot be manufactured by the human body, which is why they are called "essential" fatty acids and must be incorporated through the diet. On the contrary, the fatty acids of the Omega 9 family can be biosynthesized, so there is no need to incorporate them through food.

In the case of Omega 3 and 6, not only must they be consumed in sufficient quantities, but the proportion in which this occurs is important, since in many cases they have antagonistic effects. In this sense, while the suggested Omega6-Omega3 ratio is 4: 1 or less1, in an average western diet this value is usually approximately 10: 1, even reaching 30: 1 in extremely unbalanced cases. The risks of high concentration or consumption of Omega 6 are associated with heart attacks, strokes, arthritis, osteoporosis, mood changes and obesity, among other diseases or conditions 2, against which the consumption of Omega 3 has a beneficial effect and / or preventive as appropriate.

THE OMEGA 3 FAMILY

Within the family of Omega 3, we can find compounds such as alpha-linolenic acid (ALA), eicosapentaenoic acid

(EPA) and docosahexanoic acid (DHA), among those of greater biological importance, since they participate in the construction of the cell membranes of components of the nervous and circulatory system and contribute to improving their fluidity, flexibility and permeability properties.

Most of the ALA incorporated through the diet comes from plant sources such as flax seeds, chia, walnuts, hazelnuts and kiwis. Once ingested, it can act as a precursor to EPA in the body, from which DHA is in turn synthesized. However, this conversion is limited in its capacity and also varies between individuals, which is why it is advisable to ingest foods in which they are present, especially in the case of DHA since its synthesis involves a greater number than in the case of EPA, stages from ALA.

As additional factors, advancing age, disease and stress contribute to limiting this transformation process, while the excessive intake of Omega 6 competes for the use of the same enzymes 3.

DHA AND ITS IMPORTANCE IN HEALTH

The main benefits of DHA on the human organism are numerous and diverse, among which we can highlight:

- Pregnancy: the intake of DHA helps meet the additional nutritional needs of Omega 34. Once born, the baby continues to receive DHA from his mother via breast milk, the content of which is directly related to the amount consumed by the mother5. This is of fundamental importance, since the immediate prenatal and postnatal level of DHA has a great influence on the growth and functions of the central nervous system and, consequently, on the neurological and cognitive development of the newborn 6, 7.

- Brain health: DHA is a structural and functional element of great importance in the brain, where approximately 30% of the neurons' structural lipids are DHA. In addition to the benefits in newborns and children, DHA has been shown to help maintain normal brain function in adults, while there are scientific data linking reduced levels of DHA to a number of mental disorders such as depression, dementia, schizophrenia and alzheime8, 9, 10,11.

- Eye health: retinal photoreceptors have a high concentration of DHA where they transform light signals into neuronal activity. That is why DHA plays an important role in eye health during prenatal phase and in the first years of life7. Additionally, diets rich in Omega-3 fatty acids, especially DHA, can have a protective effect on aging-related vascular and retina pathologies in older people12, 13.

- Heart health: several scientific investigations clearly demonstrate that a high intake of Omega-3 fatty acids, especially DHA, is correlated with heart health. The effects of DHA on cardiac health include effects on triglycerides, high-density lipoproteins on cholesterol, platelet function, endothelial and vascular function, blood pressure, oxidative stress parameters, as well as pro- and anti-inflammatory cytokines14, 15, 16.17.

Omega 3 functions

Fatty acids produce a lowering effect on cholesterol and triglyceride levels, and in turn reduce platelet aggregation in the arteries. This implies that platelets circulating in the blood do not adhere to each other, thus preventing the formation of clots.

Among other functions of Omega-3, its intervention in the formation of cell membranes stands out; they make up most of the brain tissues, since the nerve cells are rich in Omega-3 fatty acids; and they are converted to prostglandins, substances with an important role in the regulation of the cardiovascular, immune, digestive, and reproductive systems and that have anti-inflammatory effects.

SOURCES OF OMEGA 3.

SOURCES OF OMEGA 6

Most of the oils that are fried (corn, sunflower, peanut)

Effects of omega 3 in type 2 diabetes and metabolic syndrome

Various investigations have proven that the consumption of omega 3 benefits patients with diseases related to an inflammatory state such as lupus erythematosus, arthritis, cancer, metabolic syndrome, diabetes mellitus, among others (16). In the case of type 2 diabetes and metabolic syndrome, supplementation with DHA and EPA has been shown in laboratory animals to improve metabolic parameters such as glucose, insulin, cholesterol, low-density lipoproteins and blood triglycerides (17, 18). They also have a decrease in the size of adipocytes, and an increase in the expression of pathway genes such as lipolysis (degradation of acids fatty) and β-oxidation (conversion of fatty acids into energy) in this same tissue (19, 20).

In the case of the liver, omega 3s have been shown to decrease the fatty liver process and regulate nuclear receptors such as the receptor that binds regulatory elements (SREBP-1) that controls cholesterol metabolism, in addition to other glycolytic pathways (21). Although there are many mechanisms and beneficial effects of the consumption of omega 3 in experimental animals, the results in humans have not always been comparable.

It is important to mention that studies in patients with diabetes mellitus, metabolic syndrome and obesity supplemented with omega 3 show variability in its effects on metabolic parameters such as glucose and on blood lipids such as cholesterol and LDL (22, 23). However, similarities have been found between humans and mice regarding some mechanisms. Studies with massive sequencing and analysis techniques find similarities in some pathways such as lipolysis and b-oxidation. However, there are other mechanisms, in addition to those already known, such as oxidative mechanisms that explain the beneficial effects on humans in these diseases (24, 25). Therefore, the recommendations suggest that the use of omega 3 acids can be used as an adjunct in the therapy of these diseases.

Effect of omega 3s on the nervous system

Regarding its beneficial effects on other tissues, it has been found in the nervous system that the increase in omega 3 fatty acids in the membranes, has important repercussions on various brain functions both during pregnancy and in early stages of development. Children of mothers who were supplemented with omega 3 during pregnancy, presented higher coordination and memory compared to children of mothers without supplementation before tests of cognitive skills (memory and coordination) (26). A study in Mexican children showed that the children of first-time mothers supplemented with 400 mg / day of DHA at 20 weeks of gestation had larger neonates and with a greater head circumference than non-supplemented mothers (27). Consumption of these fatty acids has also been shown to have beneficial effects on motor and learning functions, improved visual acuity, as well as the prevention of allergies and autoimmune diseases. (8).

International recommendations for omega 3 consumption

Due to the forcefulness of the protective effect in cardiovascular diseases, important associations such as the FDA (Food and Drug Administration), AHA (American Heart Association) and ISSFAL (International Society for the Study of Fatty Acids and Lipids) in the United States have issued recommendations for use. For the prevention of heart disease consume 2 servings of fish a week (plus or minus 300 to 500 mg / day). For patients with heart disease consume 1000 mg / day. However, they also recommend not exceeding 3000 mg / day since it could have some adverse effects such as increased clotting time and elevation of low-density lipoprotein (LDL) (28, 29). These same associations suggest that the main sources of omega 3 come from consuming mainly fish.

Although the main associations mentioned above recommend the consumption of fish in the regular diet, some researchers have warned about the high content of harmful substances such as mercury and fluorinated chlorinated substances found in many varieties of fish, which could have repercussions on health. Many of these substances have been linked to the development of diseases such as obesity. It was shown that in mice that consumed one type of Atlantic sea salmon and others that consumed salmon reduced in harmful substances for several weeks, those of marine salmon had metabolic damage and obesity, compared to those reduced in harmful substances (30). Based on these evidences and other findings, some researchers suggest that supplementation is an option to obtain the doses and the beneficial effects on health from omega 3s, but that nevertheless we must not lose sight of the origin and where they come from. These supplements.

Omega 3 interactions with other nutrients.

An important aspect to consider regarding the consumption of omega 3 are the possible interactions that these have with other nutrients in the diet. One of these is omega 6 fatty acids, main competitors in the synthesis of substances by the cell. Omega 6s are found in various high consumption oils in western societies such as safflower, corn, sunflower, among others. They belong to the same long-chain polyunsaturated fatty acids with the difference of having a double bond at carbon 6. Like omega 3s, these omega-6s are also incorporated into the cell membranes of various tissues. These fatty acids are generally associated with the production of inflammatory mediators (31). Its high consumption and its possible health implications are currently under debate.

Another of the interactions of interest is the high consumption of carbohydrates, especially sucrose, and its possible interference with the beneficial effect of omega 3. Studies show that obese rats fed high amounts of sugars (sucrose from 25 to 45 %), the animals supplemented with fish oil showed no improvement in the levels of inflammation in adipose tissue (33, 34). It is believed, derived from these investigations, that it is the simple sugars that, when consumed in large quantities, could interfere especially with adipose tissue, with the benefits of omega 3. There are so far few studies in this regard, and only in animal models. However, it would be necessary to consider the increase of carbohydrates (especially simple carbohydrates) in the diet for a better effect of omega 3.

4. FEEDING

Eat healthy and enjoy your meals!a healthy eating plan for weight control includes a variety of foods that you may not have considered. if "healthy eating" makes you think about foods you can't eat, try to focus your attention on all the new foods you can eat:

Fresh fruits: don't just think about apples and bananas. Those are great options, but also try some "exotic" fruits. How about a mango? Or a juicy pineapple or a kiwi! When it's not the season for your favorite fresh fruit, you can try frozen, canned, or dried versions of the fresh fruits you like. One caveat about canned fruits is that they may contain additional sugars or syrups. Be sure to choose fruit varieties that are packaged in water or in their own juice. Fresh vegetables: try something new. You might find that you like grilled or steamed vegetables seasoned with herbs that you haven't tried yet, such as rosemary. You can fry the vegetables in a nonstick skillet with a little cooking spray. Or try frozen or canned veggies to make a quick accompaniment, you just need to microwave and serve. When you try canned vegetables, look for the ones that come without extra salt, butter, or cream sauces. Make a commitment to go to the vegetable section and try one new vegetable per week.

Foods rich in calcium: You might automatically think of a glass of low-fat or fat-free milk when someone says you should "eat more dairy products." But what about low-fat and fat-free yogurts that do not contain additional sugars? These come in a wide variety of flavors and can be an excellent substitute for desserts for those who like sweet treats.

A healthy diet helps protect us from malnutrition in all its forms, as well as non-communicable diseases, including diabetes, heart disease, stroke and cancer.

Worldwide, unhealthy diets and lack of physical activity are among the main health risk factors.

Healthy eating habits begin in the first years of life; breastfeeding promotes healthy growth and improves cognitive development; In addition, it can provide long-term benefits, including reducing the risk of overweight and obesity and of non-communicable diseases later in life.

Caloric intake must be balanced with caloric expenditure. To avoid unhealthy weight gain, fats should not exceed 30% of total caloric intake (1, 2, and 3).

Limiting the consumption of free sugar to less than 10% of the total caloric intake (2, 7) is part of a healthy diet.

To get older benefits it is recommended to reduce your consumption to less than 5% of the total caloric intake (7).

Maintaining salt intake below 5 grams daily (equivalent to less than 2 g of sodium per day) helps prevent hypertension and reduces the risk of heart disease and stroke among the adult population (8).

WHO Member States have agreed to reduce salt consumption among the world population by 30% by 2025; They also agreed to stop the increase in diabetes and obesity in adults and adolescents, as well as in overweight children by 2025 (9, 10).

General view

Eating a healthy diet throughout life helps prevent malnutrition in all its forms, as well as different non-communicable diseases and disorders. However, increased production of processed foods, rapid urbanization, and changing lifestyles have led to a change in eating habits. Currently, people consume more hypercaloric foods, fats, free sugars and salt / sodium; On the other hand, many people do not eat enough fruits, vegetables, and dietary fiber, such as whole grains.

The exact composition of a varied, balanced and healthy diet will be determined by the characteristics of each person (age, sex, lifestyle habits and degree of physical activity), the cultural context, the food available on site and eating habits. However, the basic principles of healthy eating remain the same.

For adults

A healthy diet includes the following:

Unprocessed fruits, vegetables, legumes (such as lentils and beans), nuts, and whole grains (for example, unprocessed corn, millet, oats, wheat, or brown rice).

At least 400 g (that is, five servings) of fruits and vegetables a day (2), except potatoes, sweet potatoes, cassava and other starchy tubers.

Less than 10% of the total caloric intake of free sugars (2, 7), which is equivalent to 50 grams (or about 12 level teaspoons) in the case of a person with a healthy body weight that consumes approximately 2000 calories a day, although to obtain additional health benefits, the ideal would be a consumption of less than 5% of the total caloric intake (7). Free sugars are all those that manufacturers, cooks or consumers add to food or beverages, as well as the sugars naturally present in honey, syrups and fruit juices and concentrates.

Less than 30% of the daily caloric intake from fats (1, 2, 3). Unsaturated fats (present in fish, avocados, nuts and in sunflower, soybean, canola and olive oils) are preferable to saturated fats (present in fatty meat, butter, palm and coconut oil, cream, cheese, clarified butter, and lard), and trans fats of all types, particularly industrially produced fats (present in frozen pizzas, pies, cookies, cakes, wafers, cooking oils, and spreads)), and trans fats from ruminants (present in meat and dairy products of ruminants such as cows, sheep, goats, and camels). It was suggested to reduce saturated fat intake to less than 10% of total calorie intake, and trans fat intake to less than 1% (5). In particular, industrially produced trans fat is not part of a healthy diet and should be avoided (4, 6).

Less than 5 grams (approximately one teaspoon) a day (8). Salt should be iodized.

For infants and young children

In the first two years of a child's life, optimal nutrition drives healthy growth and improves cognitive development. In addition, it reduces the risk of overweight and obesity and of non-communicable diseases in the future.

The tips for a healthy diet during lactation and childhood are the same as for adults, although the following elements are also important:

Infants should be exclusively fed breast milk for the first six months of life.

• Breastfeeding should continue for at least two years.

• From six months of age, breastfeeding should be complemented with different safe and nutritious foods. In complementary foods you should not add salt or sugars.

- Practical tips to maintain a healthy diet
- Fruits, greens and vegetables
- Eating at least 400 g, or five servings of fruits and vegetables a day reduces the risk of developing non-communicable diseases (2) and helps to ensure a sufficient daily intake of dietary fiber.
- To improve the consumption of fruits and vegetables it is recommended incluir verduras en all the foods;
- As snacks, eat fresh fruits and raw vegetables;
- Eat fresh seasonal fruits and vegetables; Y
- Eat a varied selection of fruits and vegetables.
- Greases
- Reducing total fat intake to less than 30% of daily caloric intake helps prevent unhealthy weight gain among the adult population (1, 2, 3).
- In addition, to reduce the risk of developing non-communicable diseases it is necessary to:
- Limit the consumption of saturated fat to less than 10% of the daily caloric intake;
- Limit the consumption of trans fat to less than 1%;

• Replace saturated and trans fats with unsaturated fats (2, 3), in particular polyunsaturated fats.

To reduce fat intake, especially saturated fat and industrially produced trans fat, you can:

• Steaming or boiling instead of frying;

• Replace butter, lard and clarified butter with oils rich in polyunsaturated fats, such as soybean, canola (rape), corn, safflower and sunflower;

• Eat low-fat dairy products and lean meats, or remove visible fat from meat; Y

• Limit consumption of baked or fried foods, as well as snacks and packaged foods (eg, donuts, cakes, tarts, cookies, biscuits, and wafers) that contain industrially produced trans fats.

Salt, sodium and potassium. Most people consume too much sodium through salt (an average of 9 g to 12 g of salt daily) and do not consume enough potassium (less than 3.5 g). High salt and insufficient potassium intake contribute to high blood pressure, which in turn increases the risk of coronary heart disease and stroke (8, 11).

Reducing the intake of salt to the recommended level, that is, less than 5 grams per day, would prevent 1.7 million deaths every year.

People are often unaware of the amount of salt they consume. In many countries, most of the salt intake is made through processed foods (for example, ready meals, processed meats such as bacon, ham, salami; cheese or salty snacks) or foods that are frequently consumed in large quantities (for example, bread). Salt is also added to foods when cooked (for example, broths, different broth concentrates, soy sauce, and fish sauce) or where it is consumed (for example, table salt). .

To reduce the consumption of salt it is recommended:

• Limit the amount of salt and sodium-rich seasonings (eg, soy sauce, fish sauce, and broth) when cooking and preparing food;

• Don't put salt or sauces rich in sodium on the table;

• Limit the consumption of salty snacks; Y

• Choose products with lower sodium content.

Some food manufacturers are reformulating their recipes to reduce the sodium content of their products; In addition, consumers should be encouraged to read food labels to check the amount of sodium in a product before buying or consuming it. Intake of potassium can mitigate the negative effects of high sodium intake on blood pressure. Intake of potassium can be increased by consuming fresh fruits and vegetables.

Sugars

Adults and children should reduce the intake of free sugars to less than 10% of the total caloric intake (2, 7). A reduction to less than 5% of the total caloric intake would provide additional health benefits (7).

Consuming free sugars increases the risk of tooth decay. Excess calories from foods and beverages high in free sugars also contribute to unhealthy weight gain, which can lead to overweight and obesity. Recent scientific evidence reveals that free sugars influence blood pressure and serum lipids, and suggest that a decrease in their intake reduces risk factors for cardiovascular disease (13).

Sugar intake can be reduced as follows:

• Limit consumption of foods and beverages that are high in sugar, for example, sugary snacks and beverages and sweets (that is, all types of beverages that contain free sugars, including carbonated and non-carbonated soft drinks, fruit juices and beverages, or vegetables; liquid and powder concentrates; flavored water; energy and isotonic drinks; ready-to-drink tea and coffee; and flavored dairy drinks

• Eat raw fruits and vegetables as snacks, instead of sugary products.

How to promote healthy eating.

Diet evolves over time, and it is influenced by many socioeconomic factors that interact in complex ways and determine personal dietary patterns. These factors include income, food prices (which will affect the availability and affordability of healthy food), individual preferences and beliefs, cultural traditions, and geographic and environmental factors (including climate change). Therefore, promoting a healthy food environment, and in particular food systems that promote a diversified, balanced and healthy diet, requires the participation of different sectors and stakeholders, including governments, the public sector and the private sector.

Governments play a critical role in creating a healthy eating environment that enables people to adopt and maintain healthy eating practices.

Actions that policymakers can take to create healthy food environments include:

• Harmonization of national investment policies and plans, in particular trade, food and agricultural policies, in order to promote healthy eating and protect public health through measures aimed at:

Increase incentives for producers and retailers to grow, use and sell fresh fruits and vegetables;

Or reduce incentives to the food industry that allow it to maintain or increase the production of processed foods with high levels of saturated fat, trans fat, free sugars and salt / sodium;

encourage reformulation of food products to reduce saturated fat, trans fat, free sugar and salt / sodium content, with a view to suppressing industrially produced trans fat;implement the WHO recommendations on the marketing of non-alcoholic foods and beverages for children;establish standards to promote healthy eating practices through the assured availability of healthy, nutritious, safe and affordable food in preschools, schools and other public institutions, as well as in the workplace;examine voluntary and normative instruments (eg, marketing regulations and nutrition labeling standards) and economic incentives or disincentives (eg, taxation and subsidies) to promote a healthy diet; Encourage transnational, national and local food services and their outlets to improve the nutritional quality of their products, ensure the availability and affordability of healthy options, and review portion sizes and prices.

Encourage consumers to demand healthy food and meals through measures aimed at: promote consumer awareness of a healthy diet; or develop school policies and programs that encourage children to adopt and maintain a healthy diet;

Impart knowledge about nutrition and healthy eating practices to children, adolescents and adults;

Promote culinary skills, including in children, through schools;

Support information at points of sale, in particular through nutritional labeling that ensures accurate, standardized and understandable information on the nutrient content of food (in line with the guidelines of the Codex Alimentarius

Commission), through the addition of front labeling to facilitate consumer understanding; Y

Offer nutritional and nutritional advice in primary health care centers.

Promote appropriate infant and young child feeding practices through measures to:

Apply the International Code of Marketing of Breast Milk Substitutes and subsequent resolutions relevant to the World Health Assembly;

Implement policies and practices that promote the protection of working mothers; Y

Promote, protect and support breastfeeding in health services and the community, including through the "child friendly hospitals" initiative.

The "WHO Global Strategy on Diet, Physical Activity and Health" (14) was adopted in 2004 by the World Health Assembly. It calls on governments, WHO, international partners, the private sector and civil society to act globally, regionally and locally to promote healthy eating and physical activity.

In 2010, the World Health Assembly adopted a series of recommendations on the promotion of food and non-alcoholic beverages for children (15). These recommendations guide countries in devising new policies and improving those that are in force, in order to reduce the effects of marketing unhealthy foods on children. In addition, it has developed region-specific instruments (for example, regional nutrient profiling models) that countries can use to implement the marketing recommendations.

20 Foods to lose weight in a healthy way.

1. Avocados

Avocados are packed with healthy fats and are perfect as an ingredient in salads.

They are especially rich in monounsaturated oleic acid, the same type of fat found in olive oil.

In addition, they also contain a lot of water, so their energy density is not as high, and they are rich in other important nutrients such as fiber and potassium.

But that's not all: According to a study, people who eat avocado feel more satiated and have less desire to eat in the next five hours.

2. Cruciferous vegetables

Cabbage, broccoli, Brussels sprouts, and cauliflower are cruciferous vegetables.

Like other vegetables, cruciferous vegetables are high in fiber and tend to be incredibly satisfying for appetite.

Furthermore, these types of vegetables also contain considerable amounts of protein.

What does this mean? Thanks to their combination of fiber, protein and low energy density, cruciferous vegetables are the perfect food if you are trying to lose weight.

At the same time, they are highly nutritious and contain anti-cancer substances.

3. Whole eggs

Eggs are one of the best foods you can consume if you want to lose weight.

A study of 30 overweight women revealed that eating eggs for breakfast, instead of sweets, increases the feeling of satisfaction and causes a reduction in food consumption for the next 36 hours.

Eggs are rich in protein, healthy fats and cause a satiated feeling with a small amount of calories.

They contain an incredible density of nutrients, most of them in the yolk, and can help you get all the nutrients you need if you have a calorie-restricted diet.

4. Pulses

Legumes, like black beans, red beans and lentils can be really beneficial for weight loss.

These foods are often rich in protein and fiber, two nutrients that cause satiety and therefore reduce appetite.

However: There are many people who do not tolerate legumes, so it is important to cook them properly.

5. Salmon

Salmon is rich in healthy fats and high-quality protein and contains all the important types of nutrients.

It is a food that satisfies the appetite and keeps you satiated for many hours with few calories, so it can help you lose weight.

Salmon is also rich in omega 3 fatty acids that help reduce inflammation, an important factor in obesity and metabolic diseases.

And there is even more: Fish, and seafood in general, provide a significant amount of iodine, a nutrient necessary for the proper functioning of the thyroid.

6. Fruit

Most specialists agree that fruit is a very healthy food.

Although it contains sugar, it has a low energy density and it takes time to chew it.

In addition, the fiber contained in the fruit helps prevent sugar from being released into the bloodstream too quickly.

In other words: Fruit can be a delicious and effective supplement to a weight loss diet.

7. Yogurt

Yogurt contains probiotic bacteria that improve the function of your intestine.

This results in: Protection against inflammation and resistance to leptin, the main hormonal driver of obesity.

Whole yogurt or low-fat yogurt?. Studies show that whole, and not low-fat, dairy products are associated with a lower risk of obesity and type 2 diabetes. In addition, low-fat yogurts often contain a lot of sugar.

8. Nuts

Nuts are an excellent snack that contains balanced amounts of protein, fiber and healthy fats.

Despite its high fat content, nuts are not fattening.

Population studies have also revealed that people who eat nuts tend to be healthier and thinner than people who do not eat them.
But beware! Nuts are also quite high in calories, so watch out for binge eating.

9. Lean meat and chicken breast

Despite the fact that there are no studies to confirm this, meat has always been unfairly classified as having negative health effects.

Various studies have shown that unprocessed red meat does not increase the risk of heart disease or diabetes.

But what is the best of all? Thanks to its high levels of protein, meat is a food that helps lose weight.

Studies have shown that increasing protein intake to 25-30% of calories can reduce cravings by 60%, halve the urge to snack late at night, and cause a weight loss of nearly half a pound a day for week.

Protein is the nutrient that most satisfies your appetite, and eating a protein-rich diet can burn up to 80-100 more calories a day.

10. Green leafy vegetables

Leafy green vegetables have various properties that make them a perfect food for weight loss.

They are low in calories and carbohydrates and are packed with fiber.

Leafy green vegetables are incredibly nutritious and are rich in all types of vitamins, minerals, and antioxidants, including calcium.

Why is calcium important? According to various studies, calcium helps burn fat. Eating green leafy vegetables is an excellent way to increase the volume of your meals without increasing calories.

11. Quesillo

Cottage cheese is a food that quite satisfies your appetite, making you feel full with few calories.

It is rich in protein and contains very little carbohydrates and fat.

As it is a dairy product, it is also rich in calcium, which, as we have already mentioned above, helps in the fat burning process.

12. Whole grains

Although cereals have had a bad reputation for the past few years, some are definitely healthy.

Brown rice, o at meal, or quinoa are gluten-free whole grains full of fiber and with a considerable amount of protein.

Oatmeal is loaded with beta-glucans, soluble fibers that increase satiety and improve metabolic health.
Don't forget: Refined cereals are unhealthy, and sometimes the foods that include "whole grains" on their labels are highly processed products that fatten and harm the body.

13. Grapefruit

Eating half a grapefruit a half hour before your daily meals can help you feel more satiated and consume fewer calories.

In a study of 91 obese people, consuming half of fresh grapefruit before meals led to a weight loss of 1.6 kg over a period of 12 weeks.

In addition, a reduction in insulin resistance, a metabolic abnormality involved in many chronic diseases, was also observed.

14. Tuna

Tuna is a lean fish, so it does not have much fat. It is another low-calorie, protein-rich food.

It is popular with bodybuilders and fitness models because it is a great way to keep protein levels high and calorie and fat levels low.

15. Chia seeds

Chia seeds are one of the most nutritious foods on the planet. 28 grams of chia contains 12 grams of carbohydrates, a fairly high amount, but 11 of those grams are fiber.

In other words: Chia seeds are one of the best sources of fiber in the world.

Although some studies have revealed that chia seeds can help reduce appetite, no statistically significant effect has been found in causing weight loss.

However, thanks to their composition in nutrients, it makes sense to say that they can be useful in a weight loss diet.

16. Apple cider vinegar

Apple cider vinegar is a very popular natural product for its properties.

Various human studies indicate that apple cider vinegar is useful for people who want to lose weight.

Consuming vinegar with foods rich in carbohydrates can increase the feeling of satisfaction and, as a consequence, lead to lower calorie consumption during the rest of the day, from 200 to 275 fewer calories.

In a study in obese people: Consuming 15 or 30 ml of vinegar daily for 12 weeks caused a loss of 1.2-1.7 kg.

Vinegar has also been shown to reduce the highs and lows of sugar after meals, which can have all sorts of long-term beneficial health effects.

17. Cooked potatoes

Potatoes are a perfect food both for weight loss and for iron health.

They contain a wide variety of nutrients and are especially rich in potassium, a nutrient that most people lack and with an important role in controlling blood pressure.

According to the Satiety Index (SI), which measures satiety produced by food, cooked potatoes have the highest satiety index compared to other foods.
This means that: By eating cooked potatoes, your stomach fills up sooner and you eat less of other foods. When you

cook potatoes, let them cool for a while: they will form large amounts of starch. This fiber-like substance has all kinds of health benefits, including weight loss.

18. Soup

As we have mentioned before, low energy density foods and diets make people consume fewer calories.
Most low energy density foods are those that contain a lot of water, such as vegetables and fruits.
Some studies have shown that consuming the same food in the form of soup, rather than solid, makes people fill up more and eat far fewer calories.

19. Coconut oil

Coconut oil is rich in medium-length fatty acids.
According to various studies, these fatty acids, called medium-chain triglycerides, increase satiety and burn calories.
There are two studies, one in women and one in men, that prove that coconut oil decreases the amounts of abdominal fat.
Important: Coconut oil also contains calories, so using it as a dressing in your meals is not a good idea.
It is not about adding coconut oil to your diet, but replacing some cooking fats with coconut oil.

20. Chili

Eating chili peppers can be very useful to lose weight. Chili pepper contains a substance called capsaicin which, according to some studies, reduces appetite and increases fat burning.

This substance is also sold in supplement form and is a common ingredient in many commercial weight loss supplements.

One study revealed that consuming 1 gram of red hot pepper reduced appetite and increased fat burning in people who did not eat chili peppers regularly.

5. WHY CAN NOT I LOOSE WEIGHT?

1. EAT BIGGER PORTIONS MORE OFTEN

People eat much more outside than before. "Also, the portions now doubled or tripled, implying excess calories to burn."

2. DRINKING TOO MANY SUGARY DRINKS

A 20 ounce bottle of coca cola (almost 600 ml) has 240 calories; a starbucks coffee machiato, 230.

3. OVERESTIMATING THE CALORIES YOU BURN IN THE GYM

Without some dietary changes, exercise - while it is necessary to lose weight and improve overall health - is not enough. "Some people overestimate the amount of calories they burn when they train and don't cut enough calories from their diet."

4. UNDERESTIMATE THE CALORIES YOU CONSUME

It is a fairly common problem among people who are fighting the battle of being overweight: distorting portions. "Some studies suggest that calories are underestimated when portions are large."

5. WE ARE INCREASINGLY STRESSED

Living running, worried about fulfilling all our responsibilities does not help to lose weight. "When we are stressed our body produces cortisol, a hormone that increases appetite and leads us to overeat"

6. CHOOSE THE MENU WITH YOUR POCKET

A study from the University of North Carolina at Chapel Hill found that people eat "junk" food because of its price. If combos increase in value, then consumption decreases.

7. EXCESSIVE CONSUMPTION OF SUGAR

It comes in a variety of forms, from cookies to maple syrup, and contributes not only to increasing obesity but also predisposes to a host of health problems like high blood pressure, heart disease, diabetes and depression.

8. HAVE A PESSIMISTIC ATTITUDE TOWARDS DIET

If you are optimistic, you will feel that you can take control of your life and better influence your health." said dr. fabrizio mancini. "An optimist after going to the doctor says: the doctor is right. I have eaten a lot of junk food, i need to eat more fruits and vegetables and cut with so many calories. I'm going to start going to the gym at least three times a week. A pessimist, on the other hand, will feel unprotected, so he will never make healthy decisions".

9. Spend little time on meals

Leaving many hours without eating is counterproductive. Because hungry, we may be tempted to eat the first thing we see. Also, as explained by Dr. Jessica Bartfield, weight loss specialist at Loyola Gottlieb Memorial Hospital. "

10. Not getting enough sleep

Although it may not seem like it, sleep is closely related to being overweight. "Various studies have shown that people who sleep less than six hours have elevated levels of Ghrelin, an appetite-stimulating hormone, especially from foods high in carbohydrates or calories."

Why if I exercise I don't lose weight?

Having good eating habits and doing sports regularly is essential to obtain optimal results

This is one of the most frequent problems in the office. The main mistake that people who decide to lose weight make is that they start exercising Monday through Friday, believing that only because of this they should start to see a smaller number in the weighing machine. Let me tell you: you are totally wrong.

- The first thing they have to know is that when you start exercising it is common for muscles to swell and water to be retained, this is completely normal. Don't panic if you don't see weight changes at first and even if they increase. They must take into account the percentage of fat to see how its composition is changing, it is not only about the weight.

- The second thing to consider and that I think is the most important is diet. Don't expect to lose weight by exercising if you haven't stopped eating bad habits. If you continue to eat chips and desserts daily or if you are used to cooking everything with lots of oil at home, nothing will happen.

- Also alcoholic beverages can directly affect your efforts to lose weight. Remember that each gram of alcohol provides seven kilocalories and no nutrients. That energy does not serve the body.

- The third point is that perhaps the calories burned when exercising and underestimating the ones you eat are overestimated, which causes you to gain weight instead of losing weight.

- The general rule of thumb is that exercise will never make up for a bad diet, so if you want to make a profit, you should implement changes in both your physical activity and your diet.

IN CASE YOU'RE ON A DIET

- Cocktails with alcoholic beverages can exceed 240 calories, as can a slice of pizza.

- It is recommended to drink smoothies and shakes before exercising, since being liquid, they are easily digested.

- Aerobic movements help burn fat deposits after 30 minutes of physical activity.

- Stretching the body after being in the same position for hours helps to release tension and improve posture.

- Eat less.

- I eat well, I do sports and I don't lose weight.

It seems like a lie but eating little and starving does not imply weight loss. If you are too restrictive with your diet, what you can cause is a slowdown of your metabolism and consequently an increase in the difficulty of losing weight.

This happens by adaptation, it is survival, if we give too little to our body it must survive and consequently decides to reduce its daily caloric expenditure (basal metabolism) so that you can continue with your day to day. You must not let this happen.

To keep your metabolism agile and active:

- Eat often, about every 3 hours, healthy food.

- After workouts of more than an hour and a half add an extra snack such as a fruit with yogurt or a commercial recuperator.

Do not eliminate food groups, your meals must be complete, remember "the idea of the plate": a large portion of vegetables, a quarter of the plate of whole grains (carbohydrates such as bread, pasta, rice ...) and another quarter we will fill it with lean proteins (meat, legumes, fish or eggs).

• Perform exercise. Exercise increases the calories we consume throughout the day but something more interesting is that it helps you to increase your muscle mass in this way your body will spend more calories daily, which will help you maintain weight.

Dinner only fruit and / or yogurt

Dinner helps you regain and complete your daily energy intake. For this reason it must be complete, therefore logically eating only fruit or fruit and yogurt will not provide us with enough nutrients.

Fruit is a healthy and necessary food, but if you combine 2, 3 or 4 fruits in a dinner, the amount of sugar will be excessive and will not help weight loss.

When dinner isn't rich enough in calories or balanced:

• As we have mentioned in the previous point, if you go too little, your metabolism slows down, so there is no use in eating too little if what you achieve is to reduce your basal metabolism.

• The next morning has a bad time. If we restrict intake in one meal, it is common for hunger to be greater in the next. Consequently, if you have little dinner the next morning you will be hungrier than usual and will have a hard time avoiding snacking.

• If they have trained just before dinner, you will not recover correctly.

Eliminate carbohydrates from your diet

Don't banish carbohydrates from your meals. Always add some bread, cereal, pasta, rice or potato to have enough energy and perform well in your workouts.

Choose them whole, so you enrich your diet with fiber, vitamins and minerals, being more nutritious and satisfying.

The amount will depend on various factors such as training, height and size but at least they will represent a quarter of the plate to about three quarters.

Salads are a quick resource that we often use for our lunches and dinners. But remember that a salad is a mixture of vegetables, various vegetables, but not a mix of any type of food.

A pasta salad that has macaroni, crab sticks, tuna, cheese, and olives is not a salad because where is the vegetable?

A salad can contain lettuce, tomato, carrot, cucumber, onion, pepper, asparagus, spinach, lamb's lettuce, beets... But keep in mind that cheese, tuna, olives and sausages increase the calories on your plate.

If you fancy you can consume a complete salad as a single dish such as a pasta salad, to which you can add pasta and some type of protein such as hard-boiled egg or tuna to the vegetable base. But you will do it by being aware of what you are using, thinking about the foods you add.

Take daily high fat foods like avocado, nuts and chia seeds.

These are foods that are very fashionable, you will have read a lot about them and there are reasons to recommend their consumption. Although each one has its special characteristics, all of them provide us, in addition to a good amount of vitamins and minerals, healthy fats and fiber, this provides good satiety and consequently a correct regulation of appetite and avoiding pecking and the consumption of other unhealthy food.

If you want to lose weight and you have the habit of consuming them, it is correct, what you should bear in mind is that, being rich in fats, they are caloric foods, so keep in mind three things:

• Alternate their consumption and thus enrich your diet every day, it is not necessary that you consume them every day.

• Small amounts. A handful of nuts and a fruit or yogurt with a tablespoon of chia or toast with tomato slices and half an avocado can be a successful snack.

• Consume them at breakfast or as a snack to take advantage of their satiating effect and thus you will not want to snack between meals.

I usually consume detox smoothies and shakes

There are no miracle foods. Detox smoothies, green juices, and fat-burning shakes seem like a "discovery" for weight loss, but they may not be.

- What happens to smoothies and juices?

- If you like smoothies, they are an option to consider in your diet, but you should think about the foods you use to make them and what you want to get from them.

- If what you want is to make a snack, try not to contain more than one fruit, the rest being green leafy vegetables. You can complete it with a dairy or a drink, such as:

- A carrot, half an apple, a celery stalk, two hours of lettuce and a yogurt.

- If you want to substitute a meal, you should not use a smoothie, since getting a complete meal this way will be difficult and unnecessary. And if you are looking for a feeling of satiety it will not be a good resource either, in this case the foods that you need to chew provide more satiety.

- Smoothies and smoothies are useful before exercise, since being liquid foods are easily digested. This makes it easy for you to feel heavy when you go out for a run. You can make a smoothie before training with:

- Two lettuce leaves, a handful of spinach, half a banana, 4 strawberries and half a glass of rice drink.

- If you want the detox effect, a shake will not be the solution, the important thing is to make a healthy diet, but you can enrich your diet with antioxidants with shakes like:

- Half a cucumber, a little, 100g of pineapple and the juice of half a lemon.

- Broccoli, two carrots, half a cucumber, the juice of half a lemon and a little stevia.

- A bunch of spinach, an apple, a little ginger and water.

- What will help me lose weight?

- Your allies to lose weight.

- The tricks do not exist, nor the foods that cause an immediate drop in your weight, but some that can help your goal:

- Green leafy vegetables: vegetables such as lettuce, cabbage, spinach or Swiss chard are especially low in calories and very rich in fiber, so they add volume to your food and help you feel satiated with a very low calorie in take.

- Legumes: they are rich in protein and fiber with which they fill us, complete our food and provide few calories. Although you must watch as the kitchens! Stew and fabada will not be the best options if you want to lose weight, better cook them with vegetables or eat them in a salad.

- Dairy: if we choose them skimmed they will help weight loss, performance and health. On the one hand we have fermented milks like yogurt and kefir, which by providing dairy bacteria will help your digestions to be better, regulate your intestinal transit and the feeling of abdominal bloating that is generated throughout the day by the digestion of food. In addition, dairy products provide us with good quality proteins that can be useful after workouts, a glass of drinkable yogurt provides you with protein and carbohydrate in a good proportion, you can also consume cottage cheese or fresh cheese beaten with a piece of fruit and you will have a recuperator perfect homemade.

- Proteins of good quality: this nutrient manages to increase the burning of fat in your body, for this reason you must remember to consume them in main meals in a significant amount, choosing those foods that provide us with good quality protein and little fat, such as lean meats, fish, eggs and legumes.

- Eggs: They provide us with protein of high biological value and the most recent studies certify that they do not cause an increase in cholesterol levels or cardiovascular risks. On the other hand, if we want to lose weight, they are a perfect food: rich in proteins, they promote thermogenesis (fat burning) and provide good satiety with a low calorie intake.

- Whole grains: do not exclude them from your plate and less if you are a runner. Choose better whole (whole) cereals. You can also use foods such as oats in your breakfasts or snacks, enriching your diet with fiber and a progressive supply of energy.

- Fruits: take two or three each day. As a runner it is good for you that one is a citrus to take more vitamin C and the other is yellow, orange, red or purplish like red fruits, in order to enrich the diet with antioxidants. Finally, as a general recommendation, avoid or consume very occasionally red and processed meats (such as hamburgers, sausages and fatty sausages), fast food such as pizzas or ready meals, salty snacks such as potato chips and, of course, beverages.

Alcoholic and sugary.

6. THE BENEFITS OF DIETS

BENEFITS OF EATING HEALTHY.

Let's keep the mind awake. The brain, in order to carry out its functions, needs certain nutrients continuously, so that a healthy and organized diet allows the constant flow of these nutrients and their proper functioning.

- Helps you control weight. Eating a balanced diet with low fat and sugar content allows you to better maintain weight and keep it stable over the long term.

- Improve the responsiveness of your immune system. Since the immune system is related to a large number of nutrients, maintaining an adequate diet makes it defend itself more efficiently against foreign agents and it is more difficult for bacteria to act causing infections.

- Keeps cholesterol and glucose at bay. Unbalanced and unhealthy diets raise cholesterol and glucose levels and can be dangerous for cardiovascular health and the development of type 2 diabetes. Eating a varied, balanced and compensated diet reduces the possibility of suffering or suffering from these diseases in the long term.

- Effective to control blood pressure. a diet rich in fruits and vegetables can help you reduce problems with blood pressure and why? Those responsible are the vitamins and minerals such as potassium that they contain. In addition, people who eat healthy, tend to stay active and not practice a toxic habit, which greatly reduces the possibility of suffering from it.

- Promotes balance and proper intestinal transit. If you eat fruit, vegetables, and whole grains daily, you will have no problem covering the amount of daily fiber needed. This, in addition to improving intestinal transit and regulating its balance, reduces the risk of certain diseases such as cardiovascular diseases or some types of cancer. Remember to consume an adequate amount!

- Improves mood. Certain nutrients such as iron, folic acid, some b vitamins, and omega-3 fatty acids can influence our mood. A varied diet provides the necessary amount of these and maintains the balance of our mood, as well as a positive attitude.

Benefits of Healthy Eating

Learn about the benefits of healthy eating and the tips to carry it out. Also, find out what are the three main pillars to live healthy. Vittal tips and recommendations.

In the framework of World Nutritionist Day, which is celebrated on August 11, we share the advantages of a healthy and complete diet.

Nutrition is very important for the quality of life of people, with three pillars that help maintain good health: rest, food and exercise. The question is how to balance these three functions. A healthy diet involves consuming different food groups at each meal to achieve a balanced supply of nutrients and protein.

BENEFITS OF A HEALTHY FOOD

• Decreased risk of long-term cardiovascular disease, helping to reduce cholesterol (LDL).

• Blood pressure at normal levels.

• Reduced memory impairment and other brain functions.

• The energy necessary to carry out daily activities is obtained.

• It improves the immune system.

• Adequate calcium intake strengthens bones and prevents osteoporosis.

TIPS AND RECOMMENDATIONS

To comply with a correct eating plan, it is necessary to carry out in all cases the four recommended meals during the day: breakfast, lunch, snack and dinner.
Breakfast is the most important meal, so it will have to be as nutritious as possible (proteins and natural fibers). At lunch, you can choose foods low in saturated fat and containing omega 3 fats (for example, walnuts). You also have to replace the mid-morning meal, such as cookies, chocolates, french fries, etc., with healthy snacks or fresh fruits.
The change is noticeable when we begin to modify what we eat, choosing healthy foods and giving priority to fresh products and not processed ones, as specified by the doctor.
Most of the food consumed during the day should be fruits, vegetables, and vegetables, without neglecting meat and fish. The goal is to try to have a balance between carbohydrates, proteins and fats. Fruits, vegetables and vegetables are the ones that are going to provide us with a large part of the vitamins, minerals

and fiber, essential nutrients for the normal development of the organism.

• These products must always be steamed, grilled or baked, leaving aside frying and excess oils. Knowing how to cook saves calories and improves the taste of our meals.

• Fiber consumption is very important to regulate intestinal transit and provide a feeling of satiety, which will help to avoid consuming more calories.

• In this process, water should be the main drink, leaving aside non-diet drinks and alcohol. 2 liters of water per day are recommended.

• It is also necessary to limit the consumption of salt and sugars, since their excesses contribute to hypertension and obesity.

• Who suggests eating between 20 and 35% of total fat per day.

Recommended calories per day:
    * For an average woman, between 1,800 and 2,000.
    * For a man, between 2,000 and 2,200

7. MAKE FOOD HABITS

To eat healthy, you need to develop skills in choosing foods, the amount and the way they are prepared, for which you need to develop healthy habits from childhood. In this way it will be easier that in adult life it is no longer about tastes, but habits.

- 1. Don't skip any meal times and set your hours.

- 2. Eat five times a day.

- 3. To achieve the five daily meals you can eat vegetables between meals that is, breakfast, lunch and dinner, plus two snacks: one mid-morning and another mid-afternoon based mainly on vegetables.

- 4. Dinner at least an hour before going to sleep.

- 5. On the days that you have to stay later at school, try to take food from home or when you have to eat outside of it, choose simple, steamed, grilled preparations and avoid dishes seasoned with cream or cheese sauces.

- 6. There are no bad foods: all foods can be recommended, this depends on the ingredients and the way of preparation. For example, you can eat a hamburger with avocado instead of mayonnaise and ketchup.

- 7. If you take steps to change your habits gradually, you will have a better chance of achieving it.

- 8. Combine food! at each meal time include one food from each group, for example a fruit, a vegetable, a cereal like rice or tortilla, a food of animal origin like chicken, or a legume like beans.

- 9. Watch the portions of what you eat! The amount of food you should eat in a day depends on your individual needs, according to your weight, age, sex, and physical activity.

- 10. Choose foods that are broiled, steamed, grilled, or boiled.

- 11. Avoid fried, breaded, creamy or weathered foods.

12. Consume 6 to 8 glasses of natural water a day.

Ten tips to eat well

It is advisable to follow a series of dietary guidelines that can be highly beneficial for health. In our pharmacy they can advise us on the most suitable nutrition for us.

1. Plan a balanced and varied weekly menu.

It will help you distribute the different food groups throughout the week and facilitate shopping.

2. Establish regular meal times.

Neat schedules will allow you to eat calmly and in a suitable environment.

3. Eat five meals a day.

Breakfast, mid-morning, lunch, snack and dinner. Likewise, avoid snacking between meals.

4. Have a strong breakfast; light dinner.

Eat fruit, dairy, and toast or cereals for breakfast, to ensure full physical and intellectual performance. And at night, to sleep well, choose light foods to digest: vegetables, soups, fish or dairy.

5. Drink between one and two liters of water a day.

It is important to maintain proper hydration. Water favors the digestion of food and helps normalize intestinal transit.

6. Moderate alcohol consumption.

Wine and beer are an important source of vitamins, minerals, and natural antioxidants. However, 2-3 glasses a day should not be exceeded in men, and somewhat less, 1.5 in women

7. Avoid saturated fats, refined flours, and sugars.

Substitute animal fats for virgin olive oil, with heart-healthy properties. Choose whole foods, richer in fiber, vitamins, and minerals. And it flees from simple sugars, which favor overweight and dental caries.

8. Cook healthy.

Cook and steam, bake or grill and avoid frying and sauces as much as possible. Don't abuse precooked food.

9. Leave the salt in the salt shaker.

If you eat without salt you will protect your heart. You can substitute it for celery, vinegar or spices, and thus you will add more flavors to your meals.

10. Consult your pharmacist about food supplements.

8. FATBURNERS

Fat burners are the best selling nutritional supplements in the world today. There are many different kinds of fat burners on the market, but they all do one or more of these:

- Provide energy: most burners have a stimulant such as caffeine, taurine or creatine that increases energy levels in order to exercise longer and with greater intensity.

- Accelerating metabolism: the most important purpose of fat burners is to make the metabolism work faster in order to burn more calories and lose weight. The caffeine, green tea extract, vitamin b12 and other common ingredients in these supplements help enzymes break down food and make it more energy-efficient.

- Dissolve adipose deposits: some burners also have ingredients that help break down fat cells and expel them through the urine.

Remember to be careful with these products because there are many that have very strong stimulants that can affect the nervous system and produce side effects such as tremors, excessive sweating, migraines and tachycardia. The best option is a fat burner that fulfills these functions using 100% natural ingredients such as cranberry, apple cider vinegar, papaya, and spirulina.

Protein shakes are increasingly used and although people have to think that these are exclusively for bodybuilders and fitness people, the reality is that these shakes are wonderful for people of any age who are looking to lose weight.

We all need to eat at least 15 grams of protein for breakfast when we wake up in the morning, since by not doing so the body will have to "eat" its own reserves of protein. (it eats its own muscle), this causes the body to activate a defense mechanism that increases appetite and makes the skin saggy.

Proteins help rebuild muscle tissues that are the "stoves" where calories are burned. When you eat quality protein with the three main meals and in snacks, your metabolism stays active all day, burning more calories and helping you lose more weight. In addition to that, protein is the nutrient that has the most satiety power (it is what makes you feel most full) and thus avoid excess food or the consumption of junk food. While a quality protein shake has a satisfying power of 99%, fish has only 79% and lean red meat has 75%.

Not consuming protein has negative health effects, for women it can result in:

• Excess fat in the abdomen

• Hair loss

• Acne

• Excess hairs

• Snoring

• Warts

• Dark spots on the neck, arms and between legs

It is very important to always consume SUGAR FREE protein shakes. Do not be fooled. The shakes they consume should be without added sugar and very low in carbohydrates and sodium. Remember to always check the labels of what you are consuming.

Well family, that's it for today, I hope you liked my tips and that you apply them so that you can begin to transform your lives and say Yes I Can! If you want more information and the best advice and follow me on Twitter, Facebook and Instagram. A hug and see you very soon.

What are fat burners and how do they work?

"Fat burners are generally products made from substances such as caffeine and pseudoephedrine, the objective of which is to increase the elimination of accumulated fats by increasing body energy expenditure."

How and at what times of the day should they be taken to really be effective?

"They must be consumed before physical activity, although in reality they are not used in medicine as the main therapeutic resource to promote weight loss. Rather, they are used as a secondary, supportive resource, always accompanied by dietary and exercise indications for each patient. "

What is the time limit that can be consumed?

"That is very relative, since everything depends on each patient and each case. Basically what you should do is monitor possible side effects that these products may have on the person. In fact, these products should not have such free access to the population - as they currently do - and should not be self-medicated, because despite the fact that many of them are freely available, some have cardiovascular effects that can cause dangers to the patient, such as tachycardias. "

What type of diet should be followed so that the results are faster?

"We must be clear that a 'magic pill' will not achieve any results if there is not a good eating plan with a diet that is fractionated and low in carbohydrates to avoid the formation of lipids. This of course, must be accompanied by the consumption of enough liquid, at least two liters a day, so that not only is the consumption of these burners effective, but also the diet that is being carried out. Finally, we must not forget that physical activity must also be carried out constantly".

If someone stops taking fat burners after consuming them for a long time, is it likely that the dreaded 'rebound effect' will occur, that is, that the person can gain all the kilos that they lost?

"Eventually, there could be a certain 'rebound effect', but everything will depend on the dose being consumed. If the person has based his diet on high doses of these burners and relaxes and begins to eat more, then it can happen. On the other hand, if you consider fat burners as a supplement - as happens in medical treatments - their results may be better and less likely to lead to weight gain, if they are stopped. "

Which types of people can these remedies be effective and in which not?

"Fat burners can be more effective in people who do physical activity because their mission is to enhance the effect that exercise has on metabolism, but in reality, it is not the most important thing to lose weight. There is a lot of marketing and advertising in these products. In fact, it often happens that people consume fat burners because they are labeled as such, but in reality they are not; Sometimes these are products that only accelerate intestinal transit or that may have antioxidants, but a real fat burner is a product that somehow accelerates the body's metabolism and that produces an increase in energy expenditure and, through this mechanism, finally, the fat that is deposited is oxidized ".

What people should not take these supplements?
"Mainly, patients with cardiovascular diseases, hypertensive patients, arrhythmia problems, kidney diseases, among others."

What are the side effects that fat burners can have and in which cases can they be dangerous?

"Mainly, they can generate cardiovascular effects that can trigger an increase in blood pressure and arrhythmias, if they are consumed without a precise indication."

9. PROTEINS

What are proteins?

Proteins are molecules made up of amino acids that are linked by a type of bond known as peptide bond. The order and arrangement of amino acids depend on the genetic code of each person. All proteins are made up of:

• Carbon

• Hydrogen

•Oxygen

• Nitrogen

And most also contain sulfur and phosphorous.

Proteins account for about half the weight of the body's tissues, and are present in all cells of the body, in addition to participating in practically all the biological processes that occur.

Protein functions:

Of all the biomolecules, proteins play a fundamental role in the body. They are essential for growth, thanks to their nitrogen content, which is not present in other molecules such as fats or carbohydrates. They are also for the synthesis and maintenance of various tissues or components of the body, such as gastric juices, hemoglobin, vitamins, hormones and enzymes (the latter act as biological catalysts causing the speed at which the chemical reactions of metabolism). They also help transport certain gases through the blood, such as oxygen and carbon dioxide, and work as buffers to maintain acid-base balance and plasma oncotic pressure.

Other more specific functions are, for example, those of antibodies, a type of protein that acts as a natural defense against possible infections or external agents; collagen, whose resistance function makes it essential in supporting tissues or myosin and actin, two muscle proteins that make movement possible, among many others.

Properties:

The two main properties of proteins, which allow their existence and the proper performance of their functions, are stability and solubility.

The first refers to the fact that proteins must be stable in the environment in which they are stored or in which they carry out their function, so that their half-life is as long as possible and does not generate setbacks in the body.

Regarding solubility, it refers to the fact that each protein has a temperature and a pH that must be maintained for the bonds to be stable.

Proteins also have some other secondary properties, depending on their chemical characteristics. This is the case of specificity (its structure makes each protein perform a specific and concrete function different from the others and the function that other molecules can have), the buffering of pH (they can behave as acids or as basic, depending on if they lose or gain electrons, and cause the pH of a tissue or compound in the body to be maintained at the appropriate levels) or the electrolytic capacity that allows them to move from the positive poles to the negative poles and vice versa.

Protein classification:

Proteins are capable of being classified according to their shape and according to their chemical composition. Depending on their shape, there are fibrous proteins (elongated, and insoluble in water, such as keratin, collagen and fibrin), globular (spherical and compact in shape, and soluble in water. This is the case of most enzymes and antibodies, as well as certain hormones), and mixed, with a fibrillar part and a globular part.

Types:

Depending on their chemical composition, there are simple proteins and conjugated proteins, also known as heteroproteins. The simple ones are divided in turn into scleroproteins and spheroproteins.

Nutrition:

Proteins are essential in the diet. The amino acids that form them can be essential or nonessential. In the case of the former, they cannot be produced by the body by itself, so they have to be acquired through food. They are especially necessary in people of growing age, such as children and adolescents, and also in pregnant women, since they make possible the production of new cells.

- Protein-rich foods

- They are present mainly in foods of animal origin such as meat, fish, eggs and milk. But they are also in vegetable foods, such as soybeans, legumes and cereals, although to a lesser extent. Its intake provides the body with 4 kilocalories for every gram of protein.

- Protein in the diet .

- Proteins are the fundamental pillars of life. Every cell in the human body contains them. The basic structure of the protein is a chain of amino acids.

- It is necessary to consume protein in the diet to help the body repair cells and make new cells. Protein is also important for the growth and development of children, adolescents, and pregnant women.

- Food sources

- Protein foods are broken down into parts called amino acids during digestion. The human body needs a large number of amino acids in amounts large enough to maintain good health.

- Amino acids are found in animal sources such as meat, milk, fish, and eggs. They are also found in plant sources such as soybeans, beans, legumes, nut butter, and some grains (such as wheat germ and quinoa). You don't need to consume animal products to get all the protein you need in your diet.

- Amino acids are classified into three groups:

Essentials

• Non-essential

• Conditionals

Essential amino acids cannot be produced by the body and must be provided by food. It is not necessary to ingest them in a meal. Balance throughout the day is more important.

Non-essential amino acids are produced by the body from essential amino acids or in the normal breakdown of protein.

Conditional amino acids are necessary in times of illness and stress.

How to get a toned body

 Muscle toning consists of achieving the appearance of hard muscle when it is calm. For this to happen, it is first necessary to have the ideal weight and then, strengthen the body muscles. Once both goals have been reached, simply maintain a strength training habit that continues to harden muscle mass.

Tone up Female Body

The most common practices to tone a woman's body are different from those used by the male sex, mostly because they both pursue different goals and also have different constitutions. In women, this need usually appears with the so-called bikini operation, to mark the abdomen and get rid of sagging. But forget that using dumbbells of a certain weight makes you more voluminous. If you adjust the amount of kilos you load progressively, you will first strengthen your muscles and then begin to tone them.

Tone Man Body

The challenge of toning the body in men is usually pursued throughout the year, although in summer this practice is increased to show off very marked arms and thighs. It is true that this sex tends to carry more weight than necessary as a technique to tone the body, without realizing that this can cause significant muscle damage. With these very intense workouts, the body begins to look similar to that of bodybuilders and the muscles need a minimum time of rest before the next exercise.

Exercise routine at home to mark the body

There is an exercise routine at home to mark the body that will not take more than an hour a day. But remember that you need to dedicate a minimum of three days a week to Start these exercises, and you should do them as quickly as possible, without taking breaks between repetitions.

Butt and Leg Squats

Squats are the most helpful exercise for toning your glutes and legs. It consists of opening the legs a little more than the width of the hip, and moving the gluteus to below the height of the knee. All this with the trunk straight and the hands clasped behind the head. Holding the squat position for about 30 seconds before going back up causes more effect.

Abdominal plank exercise

There are many varieties of the abdominal plank exercise to strengthen the core. The basic is to lie down on a mat or other insulating material that you have at home, supporting only the tips of the feet and the forearms. All this keeping the body straight and above all, the abdomen firm. You will have to hold in that position for at least 30 seconds. If you notice that the body trembles, you will be doing it correctly.

Burpees routine

Starting the burpee routine is the most difficult step, but once you get used to it, you get great results in no time. You don't need any material to make it, but you do need a smooth surface floor to avoid hurting yourself. It consists of doing a squat, resting your hands on the floor and bringing your feet back with a jump, doing the flexion, getting up with another jump fully stretching your torso, and ending up slapping your head.

Bench Triceps

Bench triceps exercise is one of the most effective for toning women's arms fast. You have to place your hands on a bench, behind your back, stretching your feet as far as you can fully support the soles. Then, you will only have to lower and raise the core area, propelling yourself only with your arms. You can bring your feet closer to the bench in the first few repetitions, but the more distant they are, the better effect they will have.

Bulgarian stride or squat

For the Bulgarian stride or squat you also have to use a bench to support the tip of your foot. You have to stand in a lunge position, with your leg forward at least half a meter away from the bench, on which the tip of the other foot will rest. Once this is done, you have to lower and raise the knee of the front leg keeping it aligned with the foot. With this complete exercise you work your legs and glutes, and if you get dumbbells, so do your biceps.

Meals to tone muscles

There are ingredients that also influence meals to tone muscles. Based on the fact that you have to eliminate the intake of unhealthy fats, you have to conform to an adequate diet to achieve your purpose of having a toned body. First you will have to forget all the industrial bakery products, and those that contain saturated fats and refined sugars. And then, establish an optimal amount of carbohydrates, fats and proteins to include in your diet.

Protein-rich elements like egg white, nuts, red meat, white and blue fish, or mushrooms are crucial in the process of how to have a toned body. Also, we must have the vegetable fats of olive oil, seeds or avocado, as well as the proteins of skinned fruits, green leafy vegetables, whole grains or bananas.

Body shaping operation

We already warned that before setting the goal of having a toned body, you have to reach an optimal level of body mass. There are many people who, after having tried many diets to lose weight, fail to lose weight and need the help of aesthetic medicine. In this case, the operation to model the body par excellence is liposuction or body liposculpture.

Body liposculpture does not consist of the extraction of all the fat accumulated in different parts of the body, which good nutrition nor a large amount of physical exercise have been able to exterminate. The places where it is most common to do it are the abdomen, thighs or back, but it can be done on the double chin, hips, ankles, etc.

We consider this intervention a relief for all patients who choose it, tired of not being able to lose weight. Once recovered and with a definitive body contour, they only have to worry about toning their muscle mass, without returning to the previous situation ever again.

10 BEST RESULTS

1. Drink water, especially before meals

Drinking water can speed metabolism by 24-30% over a period of 1 to 1.5 hours, helping to burn some extra calories.

2. Eat eggs for breakfast

Eggs have many benefits, including helping to lose weight.

Replacing a cereal-based breakfast with eggs can lead to consuming fewer calories in the next 36 hours, losing weight and body fat.

And if for some reason you can't eat eggs, any other quality protein source works, too.

3. Drink coffee (preferably black)

Coffee has sometimes been unfairly demonized. When it is of good quality, it is packed with antioxidants and numerous ways to contribute to good health.

Caffeine can increase metabolism by 3 to 11% and fat removal by 10 to 2%.

4. Drink green tea

Green tea contains small amounts of caffeine, but it also includes powerful antioxidants called catechins, which are believed to work in synergy with caffeine to enhance the fat-burning effect.

Although the evidence is not entirely firm, many studies show that green tea (both the drink and the extract in supplement form) can help you lose weight.

5. Cook with coconut oil

Coconut oil is very healthy. It is high in medium chain triglycerides, which are metabolized differently than other fats.

These triglycerides have been shown to increase metabolism by up to 120 calories a day and also reduce appetite, resulting in up to 256 fewer calories per day.

The idea is not, anyway, to add it to something that has already been cooked in the traditional way, but to replace with coconut oil some of the fats that are usually used in cooking.

6. Take glucomannan

Glucomannan is a fiber that, in several scientific studies, has caused weight loss in research subjects.

It absorbs water and settles in the intestine for a time, making you feel more full and helping you consume fewer calories.

And people who take glucomannan supplements have been shown to lose a little more weight than those who don't.

7. Cut back on added sugars

Most people consume too much added sugar. This consumption is strongly associated with the risk of obesity and diseases such as type 2 diabetes and heart problems.

If you want to lose weight, you need to cut down on added sugar and high-fructose corn syrup. And be sure to read food labels well, since many supposedly healthy products are sometimes full of sugar.

8. Consume less refined carbohydrates

Refined carbohydrates are usually sugars or grains that have been stripped of their fibrous and nutritious parts.

Scientific studies show that refined carbohydrates can raise blood sugar quickly, leading to hunger and cravings, and to increasing food intake a few hours later. Consuming them is strongly linked to obesity.

Thus, if carbohydrates are to be consumed, it is better to ensure that they are to be consumed with their natural fiber included.

9. Follow a low carb diet

Extensive research shows that sticking to a low carbohydrate diet can help you lose two to three times more weight than the standard low fat diet. And, at the same time, it contributes to better health.

10. Use smaller plates

Although it sounds impossible at first glance, it has been shown that using smaller plates tends to automatically lead to lower calorie consumption.

11. Control portions or count calories

Anything that contributes to being aware of what you eat is useful. So controlling portion sizes or counting calories consumed can be a good idea, for obvious reasons.

There are studies that also show that keeping a food diary, writing down what is consumed each day or taking pictures of what is eaten, can contribute to the loss of kg.

12. Have healthy food nearby in case hunger strikes

Buying and having healthy foods on hand prevents you from resorting to harmful diet snacks.

Thus, it is ideal to resort to fruits, nuts, baby carrots, yogurt or boiled eggs.

13. Brush your teeth after dinner

Although there are no studies to support this, many recommend brushing your teeth immediately after dinner, which seems to prevent the temptation of an evening snack.

14. Consume spiced foods

Some spices, such as cayenne pepper, contain capsaicin, a component that can speed up metabolism and slightly reduce appetite.

15. Do aerobic exercise

Aerobic exercises not only burn calories, but contribute to better physical and mental health.

They appear to be especially effective at losing abdominal fat, which grows around the organs and produces metabolic problems.

16. Lift weights

One of the bad side effects of dieting is that it tends to promote muscle loss and slow metabolism.

And the best way to prevent this is to do some kind of resistance exercise, such as lifting weights. This can keep metabolism high and prevent loss of muscle mass.

17. Consume more fiber

Fiber is usually recommended for weight loss. Although the evidence is not conclusive, some research shows that fiber, especially viscose, increases satiety and helps control weight in the long term.

18. Consume more vegetables and fruits

Both vegetables and fruits have properties that make them very effective for weight loss.

They contain very few calories, but a lot of fiber. They are also rich in water, which gives them a low energy density. Also, it takes time to chew them and they provide satiety.

Several studies show that people who consume them tend to weigh less. These foods are also very healthy and nutritious, so eating them is important for reasons other than losing pounds.

19. Chew slower

It can take time for the brain to "register" that it has already eaten enough. And some research shows that slower chewing helps consume fewer calories and increases the production of hormones linked to weight loss.

20. Sleep well

Sleep is sometimes ignored, but it is as important as eating healthy and exercising.

Bad sleep is one of the main risk factors for obesity, linked to an 89% higher risk in children and 55% higher in adults.

21. Overcome food addictions

A study of 196,211 individuals in 2014 found that 19.9% of people fell within the criteria of food addiction.

If you have powerful cravings and you can't control your diet no matter how hard you try, you may be dealing with a case of this addiction.

And the only thing that works is getting help. Trying to lose weight without dealing with that problem first is almost impossible.

22. Consume more protein

Following a high protein diet has been shown to speed up metabolism from 80 to 100 calories per day.

One study showed that turning protein into 25% of the calories consumed per day reduced obsessive thoughts about food by 60%, while cutting nightly cravings in half.

Thus, simply adding protein to the diet, without restricting anything, is one of the easiest and most effective (and delicious) ways to lose weight.

23. Supplement with whey protein

If it is difficult to include enough protein in your diet, taking a supplement can help.

Research found that replacing some of the calories with whey protein can lead to a weight loss of around 4 kilos, while increasing lean muscle mass.

24. Do not drink calories (soft drinks or fruit juices)

Sugar is bad, but in liquid form it is even worse. In fact, it is probably the most fattening part of the modern diet.

For example, one study showed that sugary drinks are associated with a 60% higher risk of obesity in children for each daily serving.

This also applies to fruit juices, which contain the same amount of sugar as a soft drink. You can consume the whole fruit, but it is better to avoid consuming the juice alone.

25. Consume single ingredient foods

If you want to be a slimmer, healthier person, one of the best things you can do is consume natural, single-ingredient foods.

- Generally, these foods naturally satiate, making it difficult to gain weight if most of the diet is based around them.
- 26. Do not diet, but eat healthy
- Most diets generally don't work in the long term. In fact, there are studies showing that dieting consistently predicts future weight gain.
- Rather than dieting, it is better to have a goal of becoming a healthier, fitter, and happier person. Focus on nurturing the body instead of depriving it of things. Thus, weight loss will come as a natural side effect.

If you want to lose weight, but do not want to spend hours in the gym or torment yourself with strict diets, these tricks are for you. When you least expect it, you'll start to slim down your belly and lose pounds effortlessly!

Choose your food well.

It is not necessary to follow a diet to lose weight, but it is definitely important to make smart decisions. Avoid processed foods and choose the ones that provide the most nutrients and vitamins. You can also opt for natural and healthy foods that have a high level of satiety.

Consume fiber.

To consume fiber, you do not need to punish yourself with vegetables that you do not like, in fact, you can find it in a wide variety of foods such as: spinach, mushrooms, asparagus, broccoli, pumpkin, tangerines, plums, apples, popcorn and oats, just for mention some.

In addition, it is excellent to lose weight, increase satiety and regulate intestinal transit (forget about constipation). As if that were not enough, it is the perfect ally to reduce belly fat (lower the belly).

- Walk.
- Impossible gym routines are not necessary to slim the abdomen and lose weight, with increasing your daily physical activity will be enough: park away, go up and down the stairs, take an afternoon walk or go dancing; Some scientists even recommend walking 15 to 30 minutes after each meal to aid digestion, burn more calories, and lower sugar levels.

Moderate the intake of sugar and salt.

We do not pretend that you eat everything bland or that you do without sweets, but moderating its consumption is a good way to have a flat stomach. Why? First of all, if we do not take sugar we will keep insulin levels low and glucagon high.

Although there are other exercises to do, it's clear: sit-ups are a great way to tone your abdomen. Do you know how to do them correctly? There are many ways to train the abs. You can try:

With the typical trunk elevation lying on your back supported with the rear and hands behind, stretching the legs.

These are the two most typical and easiest exercises for people who are not used to exercising too much (seriously, it's easy to start)

As for the repetitions, you should increase progressively. Start with three sets of 15 or 20 and build up little by little.

Be constant.

And this is the key to everything. At this time of year we are always in a hurry to look cute on the beach or in the pool and we do the odd thing to lose weight. If we want to feel good about ourselves, it is best to take care of ourselves on an ongoing basis.

You have to take care of yourself all year round and not the month before our holidays. This is why:

• Play sports regularly,
• Take fruit and vegetables every day
• Drinking water abundantly should not be isolated events in our lives: they must be habits.

If constancy is not your thing, it helps your body burn excess fat in your abdomen with a fat burner of natural origin. The properties of ingredients such as L-Carnitine or green tea will help you see the results of your abdominal training more quickly. We recommend Natural Nutrition's natural fat burner, satiate your appetite and speed up your metabolism so you lose fat faster and forget about your belly. You can buy it on Amazon

Stopping eating foods high in fats, sugars, alcohol, and processed foods is the first rule of thumb to remove fat from your abdomen. Prefer to eat fruits and vegetables, lean and organic meats, so you make sure you are eating quality and low in fat. After a week, you can treat yourself to sugar or fat.

Don't skip breakfast.

This slows down metabolism and makes fat removal more difficult. Start the day with a glass of warm lemon water. Eat oatmeal without sugar and red berries. Oatmeal is rich in fiber and produces satiety for several hours.

The best way to lose fat is to exercise. Lower your daily calorie intake through intense physical activities, such as running or jumping rope. HIIT exercises are also very effective. The ideal is to start exercising before breakfast, since at this time you have not ingested calories and the body will use the accumulated calories as fuel, this slows down metabolism and makes fat removal more difficult. Start the day with a glass of warm lemon water. Breakfast oatmeal without sugar and red berries

Your diet should contain few carbohydrates. These usually distend the abdomen, such as potatoes, pasta, bread, rice, among others. Replace them with fruits and vegetables. Eliminate fat, fried, sweet, soft drinks and alcohol from your daily diet. Avoid spending more than 3 hours without trying food, since sooner or later you will binge. Eat small amounts of healthy and nutritious food in a greater number of daily meals, thus accelerating the metabolism and storing less fat.

Avoid stress. Cortisol makes you feel anxious and hungry all the time. Most of the fat you could gain from overeating will be fat that will accumulate in your belly because most cortisol receptors are located in the area of your abdomen.

Give fiber a chance. Include in your daily intake foods rich in fiber and so that it does not settle in your stomach, drink two liters of water.

Never eat a high carbohydrate load. These foods promote the accumulation of fat around the waist and in the belly, because your body remains immobile while you sleep, and there is no way to burn the calories you consume.

Avoid soft drinks, even light type. Although they do not provide calories, they make it easy for the body to store fat due to its effect on insulin. The reaction in the body is similar to that of sugar. Also cut down on alcohol. In fact, the hormone responsible for burning fat is almost completely blocked by alcohol intake. Nor is it about not being able to go out for a wine, or a cocktail, from time to time, but never in excess.

Exercising excessively in the abdomen only helps to gain muscle and make it look bigger. This is the myth that fat becomes muscle. So the solution is: exercises more diet.

CONCLUSION

A varied and healthy diet should include the following food groups: cereals, fruits, vegetables, healthy fats, dairy, meat and fish, eggs and sugar. A combination of these foods provides us with the necessary nutrients to carry a healthy diet. We need to maintain a balance so that excessive consumption of one food does not replace another necessary. On the other hand, a healthy diet should moderate the amounts consumed so as not to overtake us and thus maintain an adequate weight, avoiding this form of overweight and obesity problems.

It must also specifically to the physiological needs (age and sex) and balanced, respecting the recommended percentages of nutrients: carbohydrates around 60%, fats 25% and proteins 15%.

www.ingramcontent.com/pod-product-compliance
Lightning Source LLC
Chambersburg PA
CBHW070904250726
48662CB00003B/1503